TABLE OF CONTENTS

Chapter I
PRINCIPLES OF TEACHING AND LEARNING

A. *Why are the skills of teaching important for residents?*

The purpose of this book is to help you become a better teacher. You may be asking yourself, "Why should this be important to me?" There are two reasons. First, it is important because you do a lot of teaching; other residents, as well as medical students, depend upon you for this. According to one study in which every department within a medical center was represented, all residents had medical students as pupils, 70 percent taught interns, and 50 percent taught housestaff other than interns (Brown, 1970). Unfortunately, resident teaching skills receive little attention despite their obvious importance.

There is no doubt that the instruction received by medical students from residents is a significant part of their education. A large amount of that instruction occurs through supervision in the emergency room and the operating room as well as on the wards and in the clinics. Residents also teach medical students in Grand Rounds, Clinical Pathological Conferences, and Morbidity/Mortality Conferences. In addition, residents often make topic presentations to medical students during a clerkship. Overall, most teaching is probably the informal "modeling" which occurs within the constant exposure in the clinical services.

It is estimated that 40-50 percent of a resident's training is received from fellow housestaff (Brown, 1970). Interns and residents learn from housestaff in other departments as well as in their own. Overall, interns spend approximately 10 percent of their time in teaching, while residents spend up to 20 percent (Brown, 1970).

In addition to fulfilling your responsibilities to others, there is a second reason why teaching should be important to you. It is the best way for *you* to learn! There is a saying in education: *to teach is to learn twice.* Intuitively, doesn't it make sense that, in the act of organizing, preparing, and presenting materials to others, you learn a lot in the process? By your being a better teacher for others, we are convinced that you will be the best teacher for yourself.

B. *What is teaching and learning?*

In order to become a better teacher, it helps to have a clear picture of what constitutes both teaching and learning. This is helpful because often, in a group setting, you are *both* a teacher and a learner. Also, your work involves *both* education and service. For example, at morning report or attending rounds there may be medical students junior to you and other residents senior to you, as well as an attending physician. The previous night's admissions are discussed both to provide learning and to make diagnostic and therapeutic decisions. By understanding what constitutes teaching and learning, you can enhance the educational process that occurs in such a mixed group with mixed objectives.

To help you understand teaching and learning, consider the following statement: "If the learner didn't learn, then the teacher didn't teach." Do you agree or disagree? Picture the following cartoon strip: A little boy tells his friend, "I taught Rover how to whistle!" With an ear up to the dog's face, the friend responds, "I don't hear him whistling." The first boy replies, "I said I taught him to whistle. I didn't say he learned it."

Some people, perhaps including you, believe that if there is no learning, there was no teaching. According to this view, the verb, "to teach," is analogous to the verb, "to give." When something is given, something has to be received. Proponents of this view recognize that a "teacher" may have tried to teach, but if there was no learning, what the teacher did should not be called "teaching." The significance of this viewpoint is that we cannot say that someone is a good teacher just because the teacher seemed to teach well. What counts is whether learners learned (Machlup, 1979).

Other people believe that teaching is *anything* done by a teacher that intentionally promotes learning. According to this view, the verb, "to teach," is analogous to the verb, "to offer." When something is offered, it may or may not be received. The value of this viewpoint is that it recognizes the reality that teaching may occur under circumstances so adverse that little learning may occur. Nevertheless, the efforts deserve to be acknowledged as teaching (Donald and Shore, 1977).

We would like to encourage you to make use of *both views* in order to assess your own teaching. While the bottom line is whether, as a result of your teaching, there is learning, you should not feel useless in the absence of learning. Teaching and learning comprise a two-way process, and teachers cannot accept full responsibility for the learning of others.

C. *What are the principles of learning?*

Individuals are responsible for their own learning, especially as adults. Although educational thinking in the past has focused primarily on the needs of children, special attention is now being given to how adults learn. For example, in a handbook for continuing medical educators, the authors identified five assumptions about adult learners (Bunnell, 1980). We think these principles apply to medical students and residents as well as to the medical practitioners for which these were written.

1. Adults usually want to use what they learn soon after they learn it.

2. Adults are interested in learning concepts and principles; they like to solve problems and not just learn facts. If they participate actively in the learning process, it is easier for them to apply the concepts and principles they are learning.
3. Learning is best when adult learners can proceed at their own pace.
4. Motivation increases when adult learners help to set learning objectives. Motivation is usually highest when the subject matter relates to the immediate interests and concerns of the adult learners.
5. Adults like to know how well they are doing; feedback helps them to evaluate their own progress.

For us, the mega-principle which explains how adults, including how medical students, residents, and you, learn is that adults have to play as active a role as possible in their own learning. As stated by the noted adult educator, Alan Knox (1979), adults who seek to enhance their proficiencies see themselves as *users,* instead of recipients, of education.

D. *What are the methods of teaching?*

The importance of being active in order to learn led Whitman (1981) to develop a model for choosing and using methods of teaching which recognizes that in the two-way process of teaching and learning there are . . .

- two possible actors, the teacher and the learner;
- two modes of behavior, active and passive;
- two locations for teaching and learning, a classroom (any room where people can sit and talk) and application sites (places where people can apply what they have learned in classrooms). A two-by-two matrix is shown in Figure 1.

In the classroom . . .

- when the teacher and learner both are active, this is a *group discussion;*
- when the teacher is active, but the learner is passive, this is a *lecture.*

In the application setting . . .

- when the learner is active, but the teacher is passive, this is a *tutorial;* and
- when the teacher is active, but the learner is passive, this is a *preceptorship.*

Figure I.
Active-Passive Model

	Active Teacher	Passive Teacher
ACTIVE LEARNER	Group Discussion	Tutorial
PASSIVE LEARNER	Lecture Preceptorship	

E. ***How can you use this handbook?***

We have correlated the four methods of teaching to the *teaching you do* as residents:

Chapter II. Lectures: Consult this chapter whenever you have to make a *presentation.*

Chapter III. Grand Rounds: Residents, especially chief residents, sometimes have to plan and coordinate grand rounds. This is a special type of *lecture.*

Chapter IV. Seminars and Journal Clubs: These are the types of *group discussions* in which residents typically participate. This chapter is aimed to help you both as a leader and a participant.

Chapter V. Teaching Rounds and Morning Report: In the application environment, these are the types of *tutorials* in which residents find themselves as teachers.

Chapter VI. Bedside Teaching: In the application environment, this is the *preceptorship type* of training in which residents find themselves.

In each of these chapters, you will find two parts. In the first part, an orientation is provided which will include 1) a short discussion of the method's background; 2) an explanation of how that method fits into the active-passive model; 3) a demonstration of what objectives are best met by the method; and 4) a description of typical resident teaching activities using the method. In the second part of these chapters, five principles are provided with suggestions for implementation of each one.

Keep in mind that, in addition to the formal settings which this handbook addresses, residents are *always* teaching in an informal sense of being a "role model" to medical students and other residents. We cannot overemphasize the importance of your informal teaching.

We anticipate that many of you will use this handbook as a reference manual. In other words, when you are faced with a specific teaching responsibility, you will look up the relevant chapter. Finally, because your role as a teacher will not end with your residency training, a concluding chapter on the clinician-as-a-teacher is aimed to help you prepare for the future. Good luck — in your role as resident-as-teacher!

Chapter II
LECTURES

A. ORIENTATION

1. Background

> The lecture is the most inefficient method of diffusing culture. It became obsolete with the invention of printing. It survives only in our universities and their lay imitators, and a few other backward institutions. . . . Why don't you just hand print lectures to your students? Yes, I know. Because they won't read them. A fine institution it is that must solve that problem with platform chicanery (B. F. Skinner, 1948, p. 42).

The above passage is from *Walden Two,* by B. F. Skinner. In this utopian novel, a new society has done away with lectures. The issue raised by Skinner is whether lecturing is purely a matter of platform chicanery. According to a number of studies, we know that students' ratings of instruction are affected by the personal style of the teacher rather than by the teacher's ability to convey instructional material. This phenomenon is known as the "Dr. Fox effect." In the original Dr. Fox study, a professional actor was programmed to teach charismatically, but nonsubstantively, on a topic about which he knew nothing, "Mathematical Game Theory as Applied to Physician Education." The actor, "Dr. Myron L. Fox," was introduced with a fictitious *curriculum vitae.* He was trained to deliberately use double talk, neologisms, nonsequitors, and contradictory statements. According to almost all the 11 psychiatrists, psychologists, and social work educators who viewed the lecture personally and the 11 mental health educators and 33 graduate students who viewed the lecture on videotape, Dr. Fox used enough examples to clarify his materials, presented his material in a well-organized form, and stimulated their thinking. One mental health educator even claimed to have read the speaker's publications! *No one detected the lecture for the charade that it was.*

According to a review of the original Dr. Fox study and its many replications, Abrami, Leventhal, and Perry (1982) found that the expressiveness of the teacher typically had a large effect on student ratings, while content had a large effect on actual learning. In this chapter, we want to encourage you to focus on *both* your expressiveness or style *and* on the content of your lectures. In this regard, we could not agree more with the editors of *Change Magazine* (1978):

> The lecture is the major medium of instruction in higher education and thus the most abused. Nothing is worse than a poor lecture, disorganized and badly delivered. But nothing is more effective than a good lecture, combining substance with showmanship.

2. Active-Passive Model

Figure Ia.
Active-Passive Model for Lectures

	Active Teacher	Passive Teacher
ACTIVE LEARNER	Group Discussion	Tutorial
PASSIVE LEARNER	Lecture Preceptorship	

Returning to the active-passive model, while the teacher is active, students are relatively passive in lectures. Because the teacher is mostly talking and the students are mostly listening, lectures can be very effective in transmitting new information. Lectures are particularly helpful when the information does not appear in print. An example of information you may know which does not appear in print is your own clinical experience. By drawing on patients you have seen, you can be a valuable — indeed a unique — resource. For those of you engaged in research activities, unpublished research results constitute another example of information you have which does not appear in print. Whenever you lecture, consider including any information you have which cannot be read in a book or journal.

Of course, often you will lecture on topics that are discussed in the medical literature. When information already appears in print, you can be useful by synthesizing knowledge from many sources. This is helpful because the people you are teaching may lack the interest or the expertise to do the synthesis themselves. In fact, if they were interested and capable, they would learn more by doing the synthesis. This example is related to our earlier statement, "to teach is to learn twice." The person who synthesizes materials from many sources is going to learn a lot. When you do this synthesis as a lecturer, you probably will learn more than the students.

3. Learning Objectives

When preparing a lecture, you should clearly establish your expectations of what students will learn. These expectations are known as *educational objectives,* and, according to a model used widely by educators, there are three domains of learning or three types of objectives: *cognitive* learning refers to thinking; *affective* learning to feelings and attitudes; and *psychomotor* learning to behaviors or skills (Bloom, 1956).

Keep in mind that the learning you realistically can expect in a lecture (the educational objectives that students can achieve) is in the cognitive domain at low levels. There are six levels of cognitive learning, with each being a prerequisite for the next higher level:

1. knowledge (remembering material),
2. comprehension (grasping the meaning of material),
3. application (using material in new situations),
4. analysis (breaking material down into itsparts),
5. synthesis (putting parts together in a new way),
6. evaluation (judging the value of material).

Our view is that the lowest two levels (knowledge and comprehension) can be accomplished in a lecture. The higher levels can be modeled by the teacher, but probably cannot be achieved by students, given their passive role in a lecture.

Some lecturers try to teach *affective* objectives in a lecture, i.e., they try to teach attitudes. We think few speakers have that ability. However, there is one affective objective that should be addressed in every lecture, and that is the belief that this subject is worth knowing. We agree completely with Erickson (1980): "Most instruction involves a two-way process — presenting information while at the same time indicating its worth."

4. Typical Activities

This chapter can be consulted for a variety of lecture-type situations, including presentations to medical students in your department's clerkship and talks to nurses, physician assistants, and ancillary staff.

B. PRINCIPLES

Principle 1: *Attract and maintain atention.*

Some lectures get off to a bad start because the speaker does not successfully gain the audience's attention. A clear statement of purpose can be very helpful. Also, there are a variety of techniques that get people's attention, e.g., telling a relevant anecdote, posing a dilemma, or asking an intriguing question. After attracting the audience's attention, maintaining it is even more crucial. Research indicates that most adults in a lecture can pay attention for only 15-20 minutes before their minds wander. This is due to their passive role as listeners, in contrast to the teacher's active role as a talker. The challenge is to use a teaching technique, perhaps at the 20-minute mark, to get them re-involved in the lecture. We want to suggest three techniques for you to use: *questioning, brainstorming,* and *demonstration.*

Questioning can be used to promote thought, to evaluate what has been learned, and to move students toward your desired goals. By being asked questions, the students are thinking and therefore getting more involved. When you are asking a question, it is important to state it clearly and be willing to tolerate silence for a little while if you expect audience members to answer. Of course, sometime you might try using rhetorical questions which are not meant to be answered, but do encourage thinking.

For questions you want the audience to answer, avoid making it a guessing game. Instead, try using open-end questions that do not have a single correct answer. For example, if I were lecturing on "How to Give a Lecture," asking "How can you help keep the attention of students?" is better than, "According to the educational research, what is the average attention span in a lecture?"

Brainstorming is a special type of questioning. It is a technique which generates a wide variety of creative ideas in a short period of time. In brainstorming, the teacher poses a question and asks for as many answers as possible. Usually, it is advisable to write their ideas on a flip chart or blackboard. Criticism of ideas is not allowed, but combination and improvement of already presented ideas is encouraged. After the idea-generation stage, the teacher can evaluate the list and make the appropriate learning points. As an example, in my lecture on "How to Lecture," I might ask, "What are all the characteristics of a good lecturer?"

A third technique is the *demonstration.* By using examples, experiments, or some actual performance to illustrate a principle, you are bridging the gap between theory and practice and are providing a memorable experience. Earlier, I referred to giving a "How to Lecture" lecture. When I use questioning or brainstorming 20 minutes into the lecture, in a sense, I am *demonstrating* how to use a technique to actively involve an audience. Demonstrating how to use teaching techniques helps to keep the audience's attention more than simply telling them about these techniques.

The key to this principle is that using techniques to attract and maintain attention should be considered an investment of time, perhaps 10 minutes of your lecture, to compensate for the relatively passive role being played by the students in your lectures.

Principle 2: ***Make only one or two major points.***

"Students remember more when presented less" (Engin and Engin, 1977). Educational research indicates that some lectures are disasters when teachers try to teach too much material (Bligh, 1972).

To help you decide upon the major point you want students to learn, try the following technique. Imagine that you already have delivered the lecture you are planning. It is now three o'clock in the next morning and you go from house to house shaking students out of bed, asking "What do you remember from my lecture?" What would you want them to blurt out? It would be nice if it were more than just a fact or two. Shouldn't it be some concept or new understanding of the facts? When you are clear what is important to know, then your lecture can be organized around that theme.

Principle 3: ***Make the organization clear.***

A lecture is well organized when it helps learners bridge the gap between what they already know and what they are going to know at the end of the lecture. Many lecturers effectively provide this bridge by organizing their presentations into three parts. *First,* in the introduction, *tell* them what you're going to *tell* them. This preview provides a structure for new knowledge. Second, *tell* them! In other words, the main part of the presentation should deliver what was promised in the introduction. Third, *tell* them what you told them. This conclusion provides a review.

In making the organization clear, a handout can be very helpful. In a study of lecture notes and student achievement, Russell *et al.* (1983) investigated the effectiveness of three types of handouts: *comprehensive* handouts contained nearly word-for-word transcript of the lecture, including all of the tables and figures; *partial* handouts consisted of an outline with key tables and figures; and *skeleton* handouts had a very brief outline of subtopics. All handouts included the objectives for the lecture. Their study supported the use of partial handouts. Skeleton handouts promote *encoding,* i.e., the process by which students convert a lecturer's words into their own words. Comprehensive handouts promote *storage,* i.e., the use of notes to refresh memories at a later point in time. Partial handouts were seen as a compromise between the skeletal handouts which encourage alertness in class and comprehensive handouts which provide good summaries, but encourage passivity in the class.

Principle 4: ***Use audio-visual aids that help, not hinder.***

Audio-visual (AV) aids can be very helpful when they complement a presentation. By incorporating AV aids into your verbal presentation, you can use them to illustrate and clarify your key points. However, in general, we recommend against using AV aids for their own sake. A basic rule to follow is to select AV aids on the basis of their potential to implement specific objectives.

There is a simple explanation why AV aids can be helpful (Howe, 1977):

People generally remember . . .

20% of what they HEAR

30% of what they SEE

50% of what they HEAR AND SEE

There are many types of AV aids to choose from. For example, a flip chart or blackboard can be used to highlight key points and important terms. Photographs, filmstrips, or videotapes can be used for visual identifications. Of course, in medical education, what is the most commonly used AV aid? Slides! Unfortunately, slides are overused and abused. According to the National Medical Audiovisual Center (1976), there are three "visualizing virtues" to help you select and use slides which will help rather than hinder your lectures.

1. *Legibility:* Often, there are too many words and numbers on a slide. In general, the viewer cannot read more than 35 words. Also, the letters are often too small to be read. A rule of thumb is that letter size should be 1/15 the height of the screen. If the slides are not legible because there are too many words and numbers or if the lettering is too small, the lecturer will lose the attention of the audience.
2. *Simplicity:* Often, it helps the listeners understand the subject if information is subdivided on separate slides and if key words are used to condense the number of words on the screen. An effective technique is "progressive disclosure" which gives a sequence of slides which are cumulative. Each successive slide adds one piece of information while retaining everything from the previous slides.
3. *See/hear compatability:* What the lecturer says and what the viewers see on the screen must complement each other. However, reading slides word-for-word is boring for the audience. Instead, the lecturer should talk *about* what is on the screen. Often a lecturer may finish with a slide and begin

speaking on a new matter, but the old slide is still on the screen. This is poor see/hear compatability. Use a blank slide or shut off the projector.

A problem with slides is that often it is necessary to turn off the lights for good visibility. This also results in good sleep-ability. Keep as much light on as possible and do not plan to show slides for more than 20 minutes. Shutting lights on and off repeatedly also should be avoided because it is distractive.

Finally, talk to the audience, not the screen. Even though it is difficult to maintain eye contact with dimmed lighting, do not stop trying to reach out to your audience and communicate with them on an individual basis. A disembodied voice in a darkened room does not engage the thinking of listeners.

Many lecturers use slides to present date graphs or tables. However, Plaut (1982) points out that slides also can be used effectively to present a summary of a research design, the illustration of concepts, or to highlight the conclusion of a study. In addition, cartoons on slides can introduce a little humor. We caution you that humor should be relevant to a point you are making. As we noted at the beginning, select an AV aid on the basis of its potential for implementing an instructional objective.

Principle 5: ***Use a conversational speaking manner.***

A major principle of good speaking is to be conversational. This means using a delivery in your lectures that is natural for you. Our aim is not to change your personal style. Rather, we want to encourage you to be yourself. However, regardless of what your personal style happens to be, there still are some basic rules of conversation that apply to everybody.

Being conversational begins with looking at your listeners. By maintaining eye contact, you can help keep listeners attentive, and you can see how your lecture is being received by your audience.

Being conversational also means varying the pace of your talk. Speaking quickly through a whole lecture will make students feel overwhelmed. Speaking slowly through the entire talk will put them to sleep. By changing pace, you can help maintain attention and highlight key points. The same is true for varying the volume of your voice. Avoid being only loud or soft. In addition to varying the pace and force of your voice, using natural hand and body gestures will animate the lecture. We recommend keeping your hands *out* of pockets and trying to use natural hand gestures you use in everyday conversation.

Every study ever done on lecturing identifies the importance of enthusiasm. Students at all levels most like lecturers who show enthusiasm for their subject and the teaching of it. Of course, every person expresses enthusiasm differently. However you act when you are enthusiastic, that is the behavior we want to encourage in a lecture. Of course, if you do not like your subject matter or do not like teaching it to others, you probably cannot be naturally enthusiastic, and we cannot solve that problem.

Chapter III
GRAND ROUNDS

A. ORIENTATION

1. Background

> Once upon a time, Grand Rounds, so popular and populous that they came to be held in a hospital's auditorium or similar facility, were well organized, decorous, stately and punctual exercises. The chief and other leaders of the service occupied the front rows, and behind them, in hierarchical tiers, sat staff, house officers, students, and others. At the appointed hours, the case presentation began, and the patient's story was then unfolded, usually by a house officer or student so intimately acquainted with the facts that reference to written work, numbers, or notes was unnecessary. (Ingelfinger, 1978, p. 272).

According to Ingelfinger, Grand Rounds no longer live up to the excellence of the past. In an editorial which appeared in *The New England Journal of Medicine,* "The Graying of Grand Rounds," Ingelfinger enumerated the problems as he saw them: a progressive spiral of tardiness, spotty attendance, haltingly delivered case presentations, and a devastating din, with its most relentless component being the insistent beeper.

In response to Ingelfinger's editorial, McKusick wrote that grand rounds had not yet deteriorated at Johns Hopkins since "their presentations are viewed as the 'gold standard' . . . (and) a high standard of excellence in exposition has been insisted upon and achieved" (1979, p. 440). With this chapter, we would like to help you return to or retain, depending upon your department's current norm, this gold standard. We agree strongly with Bogdonoff, who wrote in *The Pharos,* "Perhaps more than any other session, grand rounds carries prestige and calls for the best from all participants. It has long been considered the flagship conference of a department's program" (1982, p. 16).

Your responsibility, as a resident, may be to plan and organize grand rounds for your department. In order to help focus you on the true aim of grand rounds, we have adapted the statement made by the editors of *Change Magazine* (see Chapter II. Lectures):

> Nothing is worse than a poor grand rounds, disorganized and badly delivered. But nothing is more effective than a good grand rounds, combining substance with showmanship. Although in disrepute in some circles, grand rounds is still one of the best means of conveying basic information and of analyzing, integrating, and synthesizing complex materials.

2. Active-Passive Model

Figure Ib.
Active-Passive Model for Grand Rounds

	Active Teacher	Passive Teacher
ACTIVE LEARNER	Group Discussion	Tutorial
PASSIVE LEARNER	Lecture Preceptorship	

Returning to the active-passive model, grand rounds is similar to a lecture. While there are active presenters, the audience is relatively passive. However, this was not always so. Late in the nineteenth century, attending physicians conducted grand rounds by walking through the wards and stopping at the bedside of interesting patients. When the following became too large for the wards, grand rounds were shifted to the hospital's auditorium. However, until the 1950's, it was still common practice to bring the patient to grand rounds at which time the intern made a case presentation. The patient was questioned by senior physicians. After the patient left, a staff member initiated discussion.

Even if it is not convenient to bring the patient to grand rounds, we recommend a return to the more interactive model of the past. Instead of using a patient's history to introduce a general topic review, we suggest that the history be used to provide a focus for discussion and to encourage audience members to become actively engaged in problem solving.

3. Learning Objectives

In Chapter II, we expressed the view that most lectures should aim at the two lowest levels of cognitive learning, i.e., *knowledge* and *comprehension.* As a variation of the traditional lecture, grand rounds should be seen as an opportunity to achieve higher level objectives, including *application, analysis, synthesis,* and *evaluation.* At the very least, the presenters should *model* these higher level objectives. In other words, grand rounds should provide an opportunity for attending physicians and consultants to share what their thinking was in the course of the case being presented:

- What was new or unique about this patient's care that would be *applicable* to the care of future patients?
- How did they *analyze* the specifics of the patient's problem?
- How did they *synthesize* the many pieces of data?
- How would they *evaluate* the diagnosis and treatment in retrospect?

In other words, in grand rounds, speakers should think aloud rather than merely recite facts. Of course, in a truly successful grand rounds, audience members will be encouraged to think along as well.

4. **Typical Activities**

In your department, there probably is a weekly or monthly grand rounds schedule. Often, only the chief resident is assigned to plan and organize the presentations. However, all residents should consider using the grand rounds format for special lecture presentations such as clinical pathology conferences and morbidity/mortality conferences.

B. PRINCIPLES

Principle 1: ***Select a case which is important.***

In a survey of chief medical residents, Bogdonoff (1982) found that basic sciences topics and reviews of fundamental pathophysiologic processes received the major emphasis in grand rounds. According to his survey, there is a relative underemphasis on the psychological, behavioral, and economic aspects of medical care. Bogdonoff concluded,

> It seems that, overall, medical grand rounds is predominantly a forum for didactic presentations at which individual patients are frequently seen and interviewed and where patients' personal attitudes, feelings, and social problems received little or no specific attention (p. 18).

Regardless of your specialty, we want to encourage you to plan a grand rounds which is focused on a patient problem. Also, while we are not recommending that every grand rounds focus on behavioral issues, we are suggesting emphasis on comprehensive discussions which highlight the interconnectedness of physical, psychological, social, and economic problems.

The key to achieving the "gold standard" in your grand rounds will be to begin with a specific patient case that is topical, interesting, and challenging. Ask yourself, "What is there about this case that highlights an important issue in diagnosis or management?" If you cannot think of an important issue, you have chosen a poor case.

Principle 2: ***Select a speaker who is knowledgeable and interesting.***

In any given patient case, several individuals probably are involved. Be selective regarding which speaker(s) you invite. Besides selecting people who are knowledgeable, your obligation extends to selecting people who also are interesting. Perhaps as an intern you should begin planning for the day when you will have to schedule grand rounds. We strongly recommend that you keep a personal record of the many speakers you hear in the course of your training program. One technique which can help you keep track of speakers is to fill out an index card for every speaker you hear. On one side of the card, summarize what you learned about the person's expertise. By jotting down the topic you have heard and how knowledgeable the person seemed, you will be able to build up a network of experts. Also, when you interact with staff in the course of daily patient care, you can add topic areas on their index cards. On the other side of the card, jot down a few comments about the person's presentation skills. Was this person interesting? . . . organized? . . . stimulating? Thus, you will have a record of who is *both* knowledgeable and speaks well.

Principle 3: ***Orient speakers to discuss, not lecture.***

Often, when residents ask attending physicians to speak at some event, like grand rounds, they are so concerned with *getting* a speaker that they are reluctant to prepare him/her. Although it is natural to be so thankful that someone will make a presentation that you shy away from being directive with that person, we suggest that you are doing *both* the speaker and the audience a favor by making clear your expectations.

Let the speaker know that audience participation is desirable. Encourage your presenter to ask questions of the audience and to welcome *their* questions. Prompt speakers to pose problems for the audience to consider or to present alternatives in diagnosis or treatment for participants to ponder. Suggest to presenters that a conversational manner is desirable as is maintaining eye contact with the audience. Also, let the speaker know something about the audience, e.g., its size and composition.

Principle 4: ***Present sufficient data to identify, but not solve problems.***

Audience members need the relevant parts of the patient's history, physical examination, laboratory, and x-ray results. The key is to withhold until later in the presentation results that will reveal the final diagnosis and treatment needs. In a successful grand rounds, the audience participates mentally in solving the patient's problems.

The introductory case presentation should be only *five minutes* long. The pertinent data and key points should be on a handout with places for audience members to write and take notes. *Never* read the presentation. This is incredibly boring! Instead, highlight the key points in the handout.

Principle 5: ***Elicit audience participation.***

The resident should take responsibility for controlling the flow of presentations. After opening with the case presentation, introduce the speaker(s). Let the audience know that their questions and comments are not only welcome, but that they are essential to the success of grand rounds.

If a series of speakers is scheduled, use the transitions between each speaker to elicit open participation from the audience. Do they have questions? What is their opinion of the diagnosis offered? How would they have managed the patient? The resident can play a key role in setting these ground rules and keeping track of the time. At the end, the resident definitely should ask for an evaluation of the patient case. What would audience members have done differently? What principles would they apply in future cases?

You, the resident, must keep in focus that a grand rounds is more than a lecture on a topic. It is a problem-oriented and problem-solving exercise *for the audience.*

Chapter IV
SEMINARS AND JOURNAL CLUB

A. ORIENTATION

1. Background

A story is often told about Woodrow Wilson's days as a distinguished Princeton professor. Wilson strode into a graduate student seminar and abruptly opened class by asking, "Any questions?" When no questions were asked, he picked up his papers, announced that class was over for the day and left the room, apparently satisfied that no further teaching was necessary.

In this chapter, we will provide you with skills that will help you be a bit more facilitative in seminars and other types of group discussion sessions than was Woodrow Wilson. The story illustrates well both the potential value and the inherent danger of using group discussion as a teaching format. On the one hand, students who are motivated and curious, and have the opportunity to ask questions and actively interact with other students and the teacher, are likely to achieve learning objectives beyond those of knowledge and comprehension. They will be able to apply and analyze the material being taught. On the other hand, a poorly led discussion, in which the format is unclear, the teacher or students are unprepared, and the atmosphere dull or strained, is worse than a poor lecture. Since the students' expectations are greater, the missed learning opportunities are therefore more disappointing.

Seminars, of which research seminars and journal clubs are examples, are group discussions of the most pure sort. A group discussion can be characterized according to whether it is based on the needs and skills of the teacher, the learner, or the entire group (Whitman and Schwenk, 1983 p. 11). In this case, seminars would be an example of a teacher-centered discussion, in which —

- the amount of leadership required of the teacher is *high;*
- the degree of responsibility by the teacher for the outcome is *high;*
- the amount of reinforcement of the learner required of the teacher is *high;*
- the previous level of subject knowledge required of the learner is *low;*
- the dominant style of interaction of the group is *teacher-directed;* and
- the specific teaching technique used is *questioning.*

We imagine that most activities of this kind will be led by a senior resident, for the benefit of junior residents. However, this type of teaching can accommodate learners of all levels, from that of a junior medical student sitting in on a resident teaching seminar, to that of a senior faculty member with extensive research accomplishments participating in a research seminar. Whatever the background level of knowledge of the participant, a common characteristic must be a motivation to learn and a willingness to actively participate. If this condition exists, learning can comfortably occur at the appropriate level for each participant, including the teacher.

Just as a group discussion has certain distinct characteristics, so does the discussion leader. We hope that, in most cases, the resident will take primary responsibility for the conduct and outcome of the session, even if faculty members are present. Therefore, we will describe characteristics as if the resident *is* the teacher. There are three particularly important characteristics of the successful discussion leader:

a) the teacher should demonstrate, through word and action, a willingness to *encourage participation* by the learners;

b) the teacher should have a *capacity for professional intimacy* with the learners; and

c) the teacher should have the ability to *control the tension level* of the session (Whitman and Schwenk, 1983 p. 6).

We will provide help later in this chapter for you to become proficient in these skills.

2. Active-passive Model

As has been previously described, a group discussion is a learning experience when both teacher and learner are active (Figure Ic).

Although the teacher maintains responsibility for the conduct and outcome of the session, the learner must actively participate in the question-and-answer format in order to benefit. Should the learner be passive (and the teacher allow that to continue), the session reverts to a lecture, and intended learning objectives will not be met.

3. Learning Objectives

In the hierarchy of learning objectives described earlier, the group discussion method is appropriate for the accomplishment of higher order cognitive objectives and, occasionally, affective objectives. While lectures are best at transmitting *knowledge* and modeling *comprehension,* group discussion is best for learning *application, analysis,* and *synthesis* of the subject material. The essentials of fluid and electrolyte physiology are best transmitted through lecture;

Figure Ic.
Active-passive Model for Seminars and Journal Clubs

	Active Teacher	Passive Teacher
ACTIVE LEARNER	Group Discussion	Tutorial
PASSIVE LEARNER	Lecture Preceptorship	

an understanding of the application of this physiology to writing post-operative intravenous fluid orders in an abdominal surgical patient is better achieved with group discussion. The pharmacology of adrenergic receptor blocking medications is best taught with a lecture; the understanding of the somewhat unclear use of beta-adrenergic receptor blocking drugs in the post-myocardial infarction patient is better accomplished with group discussion. Group discussion is also a helpful format for the learning objective of *evaluation,* such as in the critical review of recent research. Finally, certain *affective* learning objectives may be accomplished, particularly when a group has worked together over time, and the professional attitudes of the teacher become those of the learners.

4. Typical Activities

Examples of resident teaching activities for which group discussion would be appropriate include *resident seminars* and *noon teaching sessions,* which are usually the responsibility of the chief resident; *research seminars,* where residents and fellows might present their work and that of others for critique; *journal club,* which may be a rotated responsibility; *preclinical medical student discussion groups,* which are often used as an adjunct to the basic science lectures of the preclinical years; and *senior medical student clerkship discussion groups,* such as those which might be run by a chief resident on a weekly basis throughout a clerkship rotation.

B. PRINCIPLES

Principle 1: *Prepare for the group discussion as much as, or more than, you would for a lecture.*

Many studies have shown that excellent teachers, when asked how much preparation time they devote to a lecture vs. that for a group discussion, report giving significantly less time to the latter. This is unfortunate because the difficulty of conducting a spirited, participative discussion demands that the teacher be even more prepared than for a lecture. The teacher should, of course, be as knowledgeable about the material as possible. This includes delving into deeper levels of content that may be uncovered by particularly probing questions, or at least being familiar with current sources where answers may be found in follow-up. A list of questions should be prepared in advance, questions that are open-ended and divergent (more about that later), and designed to stimulate curiosity or encourage higher levels of learning. Listing possible answers or solutions and anticipating areas of confusion or difficulty are helpful. The teacher should also prepare cases, examples, anecdotes, or "war stories" to make the material more relevant to the learners' experience. For example, relating the experience of personally managing an out-of-hospital cardiac arrest in a spectator at a football game is certain to stimulate questions about one-man cardiopulmonary resuscitation technique. In summary, being prepared with two or three times the necessary amount of facts, cases, and stories will ensure a discussion that is rich for the learners and minimally anxious for the teacher.

Principle 2: *Set "ground rules" for the group.*

The teacher should make sure the topic is clear, well-defined, and appropriately limited. It should be as real and relevant to the learners' experience as possible. The teacher should make clear that a lecture will not be given and that participation is not only necessary for the learners to learn, but may affect their grade or evaluation as well. This is an example of the shared responsibility for outcome mentioned earlier. The teacher should set a clear norm for participation by knowing the learners by name and facilitating necessary introductions, including, perhaps, learning a bit about the background of each participant. Arranging the seating in a circle, so that all participants can see each other, is also helpful. Finally, the time requirements of the session must be defined. Enthusiastic participation is rarely possible for more than one hour.

Principle 3: *Encourage participation.*

The teacher's armamentarium includes the use of silence, open-ended questioning, paraphrasing, encouragement, summarizing, and mild amounts of challenge or evaluation. In general, all comments and questions are welcome, and any discussion is better than no discussion. The teacher must be comfortable with silence, giving learners a chance to organize their thoughts before speaking. Direct questions should usually be open-ended and divergent. Open-ended means that a single short answer is impossible. *Divergent* means that a question will have several (at least partially) right answers that lead to further questions and discussion. Rephrasing the question may be necessary if it is met with blank stares, but the teacher should not be too hasty. Providing positive feedback and focusing on the "correct" part of a complex answer will encourage further discussion. Clinical problems often have several correct alternative solutions, and making this fact explicit will encourage discussion (not to mention teaching an important problem-solving concept in medicine). Summarizing the answers and thoughts on a problem or topic and asking about the next step is often helpful. The teacher should use judicious amounts of challenge (the "devil's advocate" role) to confront learners with inaccuracies or inconsistencies, but this requires a level of trust, mutual understanding, and professional collegiality (professional intimacy) that may not develop for several sessions. Humor (not ridicule or sarcasm) may help here.

The primary role of the teacher in a group discussion is to be the gatekeeper or moderator that controls both the participation and emotional tone of the learners. For the quiet learner not participating, the teacher should ask direct, but gentle, questions and should pay attention to non-verbal signals of the learner who might contribute if given a little room. The teacher should also avoid always looking directly at the learner who is speaking, so as to discourage the development of a limited two-party conversation. For the excessive talker, involving others may provide balance, but occasionally a direct confrontation, preferably outside of class, is necessary.

Principle 4: *Deal appropriately and constructively with difficult situations.*

Some topics generate considerable emotion, such as care of the dying patient or the alcoholic, and the teacher must model appropriate professional attitudes, while still acknowledging and dealing with negative or unpleasant feelings. Careful paraphrasing of the emotional content of a learner's statement is often helpful. Conflicts between teacher and learner, or among learners, often arise, but these can be excellent learning opportunities if handled correctly. First, the conflict needs to be acknowledged by the teacher, thus giving it legitimacy. The teacher can then ask for a further definition of the conflict, followed by supportive data or arguments. A list of advantages and disadvantages of a particular therapy might be generated. A cost-benefit analysis could be made. If necessary, further research, such as library reading, could be assigned and the conflict resolved at the next session. Finally, some learners are so uncomfortable with the group process that they challenge the process and teacher directly. Tact is required to understand the underlying "agenda" of this challenge and constructively respond to it, while still meeting the learning needs of others.

Principle 5: ***Bring to closure both the group process and the learning objectives.***

Just as a good group discussion needs a clearly defined beginning, it needs a similar end. The teacher should acknowledge and commend the positive contributions of each participant. The content and conclusions of the discussion should be summarized, with necessary clarifications. Alternative solutions should be mentioned, and any assignments for future work that were made should be reiterated. The final comment should perhaps be an evaluation by the teacher of the adequacy of the group process itself, pointing out areas of possible improvement and ending on an optimistic tone regarding the anticipation for even greater excitement in the next session.

Chapter V
TEACHING ROUNDS AND MORNING REPORT

A. ORIENTATION

1. Background

Do your teaching rounds, work rounds, or morning report seem like any of these examples?

a) The attending is well-known for arriving late and leaving early for morning report, due to his own research and clinical demands. Knowing this, the admitting resident presents the most complicated patient admission first. As the resident finishes his presentation, the attending makes a few superficial remarks and abruptly leaves rounds to the supervision of the chief resident.

b) During the course of the case presentation, every resident is paged and on the telephone for at least part of the presentation so that by the end no one can discuss the entire case.

c) After the case presentation is finished, two senior residents get into a heated argument about the use of a particular drug, and the argument carries on so long that several residents leave to finish writing morning orders.

The obvious point is that, like most of graduate medical education, there are often strong conflicts in teaching rounds between patient care needs and educational objectives. Unlike many other activities, however, the balance seems to frequently weigh too heavily toward service needs, to the detriment of educational needs. Our opinion, and what we will help you accomplish in this chapter, is that, in most circumstances, the "work" of work rounds can be accomplished comfortably, and *simultaneously,* with the educational work. While the intern is attempting to generate a differential diagnosis, the chief resident wishes to teach brainstorming and deductive reasoning. While the residents struggle with caring for a critically ill patient, the supervising resident is demonstrating the ability to critique and modify previous treatment decisions and modeling the behaviors of a mature and seasoned attending physician. The point is that the activities and outcomes of day-to-day patient care not only can, but must, co-exist pleasantly with the teaching of clinical problem solving and decision making. We recognize that the main purpose of a particular set of rounds may be more for work in some cases, and more for teaching in others. Flexibility in this regard is helpful, while attempting to meet at least a few objectives of both patient care service and teaching.

So what role does the teacher-resident play in these rounds? The resident has responsibility for assuring that both patient care and educational objectives are met. He/she may, at different times, play the role of presenter, discussant, or facilitator and should try to be comfortable moving from one to another. The presence or absence of an attending physician or faculty member does not generally alter the role, and the supervising resident should feel comfortable in keeping rounds within certain time constraints, no matter who is speaking. Fortunately, you, and not we, have to deal with your Chief of Service in this regard. We would note, however, and will emphasize in Chapter VII, that all faculty can benefit from the teaching done by senior residents, especially in the area of current clinical literature. We would encourage you to take your responsibility for teaching your faculty seriously.

2. Active-passive Model

Teaching rounds and work rounds are somewhat like a tutorial with some characteristics of a group discussion. Specifically, the teacher might be relatively more passive and the learners relatively more active.

Figure Id.
Active-passive Model for Teaching Rounds and Morning Report

	Active Teacher	Passive Teacher
ACTIVE LEARNER	Group Discussion	Tutorial
PASSIVE LEARNER	Lecture Preceptorship	

In this blend of tutorial and group discussion, the amount of leadership required is *low to medium*, the degree of responsibility by the teacher for the outcome is *low to medium*, and the amount of reinforcement of the learners required of the teacher is *low to medium.* These three characteristics are inversely related to the previous level of knowledge required of the learners, which is *medium to high.* For example, if the housestaff assigned to a particular ward one month have an especially *high* level of previous knowledge, the amount of leadership, degree of responsibility, and amount of reinforcement required of the chief resident will be *low.*

3. Learning Objectives

As we have already mentioned, higher order cognitive objectives and affective objectives are best accomplished with tutorial and group discussion techniques in teaching/work rounds. These objectives include *analysis, synthesis, evaluation,* and changes in professional demeanor or *affect.* Specifically, the types of purposes that are best met by this method are to learn *independent reasoning* and *clinical judgment,* to learn *effective communication* of *clinical material,* and to learn the art of *critique* and *clinical consultation.* While this teaching style would not be appropriate for transmitting certain facts about the anatomy of the peritoneal cavity, it is perhaps the best way of teaching how to evaluate and manage a patient with abdominal pain.

4. Typical Activities

We have described the usual types of rounds to which these teaching skills apply. They include *morning report, resident work rounds* and *team conferences, attending work rounds,* and *Chief of Service rounds.*

B. PRINCIPLES

Principle 1: *Establish an efficient format that satisfies time constraints.*

The easiest way to fail in meeting the educational objectives of teaching rounds is to take so long in doing so that the admitting residents mentally (or physically) leave rounds in order to get their daily work done. It is the supervising resident's responsibility to determine the number of patients to be presented or discussed and to verbally commit to finishing at a specified reasonable time. A simple statement to this effect at the beginning of rounds is helpful. Contrary to popular thinking in medical education, more is rarely better. An efficient and succinct approach to each patient, in which important, but not necessarily all, points are highlighted, is clearly the most productive, both for patient care and learning. Completeness, at the expense of clarity and significance, is *not* to be encouraged.

We would strongly suggest that patients be presented in the well-known SOAP format, even those presented briefly in follow-up. Only pertinent positive and negative points should be included, so that even the most complicated patient can be presented in no more than *five* minutes. Again, significance is more important than completeness. While you are all familiar with the content of a standard SOAP presentation, we wish to highlight the following points. Historical information should focus almost solely on the chief complaints, with only *very* pertinent past history and systems review included. A modest amount of social history is helpful, so as to give others a mental image of the patient. This information will also usually figure preminently in patient management and disposition. Only *pertinent* aspects of the physical examination should be reported. The reporting of obscure signs, especially with eponyms, is to be discouraged. The reporting of laboratory findings should include a justification of costs and risks. The diagnostic assessment should include specific hypotheses, in the form of a problem list, and should include a defense. The clinical reasoning should be made explicit and apparent. The management plan should acknowledge acceptable alternatives.

An efficient format is one that balances the conflicting time needs of patient care (less time) and teaching (more time), while giving learners sufficient physical comfort to encourage their participation. Most new patients can be adequately discussed in 10 or 15 minutes, previously admitted patients in much less. The room should have comfortable and adequate seating, and allow each participant to see all others. Rounds in which the medical students stand uncomfortably in the back, or in which the entire group walks, as if with some vestigal memory of Oslerian days, are rarely productive. The description of these rounds as a "mass of shifting dullness" is an apt one. If bedside teaching or examination is required, it is better handled at a different time, usually with a smaller group (see Chapter VI).

Principle 2: ***Work to prevent dominance of the discussion by yourself or others.***

Repeat the following phrase three times: "Teaching rounds are not lectures." A well-known phrase, attributed to A. Bronson Alcott in *Orphic Sayings,* is that "the true teacher defends his pupils against his own personal experience." In other words, the paradox for the teacher is to use his/her influence to make the students independent of that influence. An important goal of teaching rounds is to teach the process of clinical decision making and problem solving. In order for this learning to occur, it seems logical that students need to do a little work, to venture guesses and opinions, to ask questions, and to challenge others. These things will not happen if only one or two participants do all the talking. The role of the supervising resident, then, is to guarantee equal access to "air-time" for all concerned. A student (or faculty member) dominating the discussion should be thanked for the contribution and a direct, open-ended question asked of a less participative member. The expectation should be created at the outset that all contributions of a genuine effort are not only tolerated but welcome. The leader of rounds must have a fair degree of tolerance for ambiguity of purpose and direction to allow exploration and experimentation. As noted by Rubeck and Pratt, what is most important is "a degree of restraint which prevents leaders from imposing their own reactions, thoughts, values, and behavior on other participants" (1978 p. 2). This requires of leaders "a willingness to wait, while others attend to, interpret, and respond to the discussion in their own perceptions, thoughts, and manner of communication" (p. 2).

In summary, before we deal with specific discussion techniques, the role of the teacher is to —

- set the time constraints of the session,
- arrange the room to encourage discussion,
- create an expectation of discussion and learner-centered teaching,
- avoid lecturing or answering too many questions directly,
- ask questions that encourage further probing, and
- never interrupt productive discussion.

Principle 3: *Use open-ended, divergent questions as the dominant mode of teaching.*

If the supervising resident provided few actual answers, but asked mostly questions that had no single, short answers, the teaching rounds would be a guaranteed success. As noted by Rubeck and Pratt, questions should be asked such that "the respondent must not only recall factual information, but also manipulate it, discriminate the relevant aspects, assemble the facts, factors, and thoughts, and judgments into a pertinent response. In responding to such 'higher level' questions, the student relates facts, makes comparisons, gives explanations, predicts consequences, or makes conclusions" (1978 p. 3). Asking the student the normal range of serum sodium concentrations is relatively boring and educationally less useful. Asking a student the significance, and likely cause, of a serum sodium of 160 mg% in a nursing home patient is far more productive.

The types of questions which promote this type of thinking are those which are *open-ended,* meaning that short answers are insufficient, and *divergent,* meaning that there is more than a single, correct answer. Students should be asked to *clarify, support, defend, justify, correlate, critique, evaluate, analyze, interpret,* and *predict.* They should *not* be asked to state facts or answer "yes or no."

The following are examples of questions that will promote discussion:

- Based on the history to this point, what diagnoses are you considering?
- Based on this history, what physical findings will you be particularly looking for?
- What is the significance of the physical finding just presented?
- Given the physical examination, how is your original differential diagnosis altered?
- Based on this history and physical examination, what laboratory tests are indicated?
- How would you justify the use of ______________ test?
- What would you do if ______________ test were unavailable?
- Do you think this patient should have been admitted? Why or why not?
- What alternatives for treatment are there?
- What do you think of the treatment proposed by the presenter?
- What are the critical factors to monitor in the next ________ hours/days?
- What should be done for this patient after he/she leaves this hospital/office?

As the discussion widens, the facilitator should gradually bring it to closure by asking more directed and closed questions, similar to techniques of patient interviewing. In this open/closed, accordion-like fashion, many ideas are generated and the best agreed upon, generating interest and enthusiasm for all participants.

Principle 4: ***Promote the ability of clinical problem solving as a goal.***

An ideal goal of teaching rounds is to teach the art of clinical problem solving and decision making at the same time that actual problems are solved and actual decisions made. The role of the experienced supervising resident is crucial to the achievement of this educational goal. Of greatest help will be the ability to make the clinical reasoning process visible, apparent, and explicit, rather than hidden and nebulous as is often the case. *The critical factor is that clinical reasoning is a deductive, rather than an inductive, process.*

Scientific investigation and research is an inductive process, in which massive data are collected and an explanation or hypothesis springs, almost magically, from well-trained intuition. Clinical decision making, on the other hand, is a deductive process in which empirically tested paradigms directly link hypotheses to even a single piece of datum, such as a physical examination finding or laboratory test result. The experience of the supervising resident must be made apparent in this process. When the chief surgical resident hears of a patient presenting with painless hematuria, the decision to evaluate a genitourinary cancer should be made explicit so that students understand why that diagnosis, and not infection, is first on the list. Similar comments can be made about the findings of painless jaundice, pediatric periumbilical pain, or amenorrhea in a female of reproductive age. The teacher's vast store of clinical experiences must be made visible and relevant to the learner. As noted by Elstein *et al.*, "The differences between experts and weaker problem solvers are more found in the repertoire of their experiences, organized in long-term memory, than in differences in the planning and problem-solving heuristics employed" (1978 p. 276). In other words, maximal learning will occur when learners struggle energetically with a difficult clinical problem, guided with illuminating questions and well-timed clinical "pearls."

Principle 5: *Bring closure to both patient management issues and the teaching process itself.*

As we have said, teaching rounds often have both patient care and educational objectives. The accomplishment of one without the other is a hollow victory. At the end of each patient presentation, the teacher should make a definite statement regarding the adequacy of the data collected, the diagnosis(es) finally agreed upon, and an appropriate diagnostic and therapeutic plan. Patient care should not suffer from the ambiguity of the learning process. At the same time, however, the teacher can also comment on the quality of patient presentation, the legitimacy of alternative diagnoses offered, the originality and cost-effective nature of the laboratory evaluation, and the accuracy of the initial treatment plan. Assignments for further reading or data collections can be reiterated, and the quality of the overall discussion can be critiqued.

Indications of success in the tutorial process are the presence of certain learner behaviors, such as the student noting inconsistencies or inaccuracies in the material presented, citing relevant information from current literature, asking insightful questions, offering comments freely, and indicating personal opinions clearly and freely (Rubeck and Pratt 1978). Another excellent indicator, by the way, is that everyone had a chance to talk!

Chapter VI
BEDSIDE TEACHING

A. ORIENTATION

1. Background

There is no better way to introduce the subject of bedside teaching than with a quotation from Sir William Osler, who noted that there should be "no teaching without a patient for a text, and the best teaching is that taught by the patient himself" (Osler, 1903, p. 50). In the early 1900's, as a revolution in medical education was occurring in which a scientific basis for medical practice was being developed and taught, Osler recognized the critical need for an increased emphasis on providing practical bedside experiences for students and residents "to educate the eye to see, the ear to hear, and the finger to feel" (Osler, 1903, p. 50). This contrast between the technological and personal aspects of medical practice and education would seem to be even more dramatic today. The explosion in biomedical knowledge, and in concommitant diagnostic and therapeutic technologies, does not at all obviate the need for teaching *about* patients, *with* patients, and even *by* patients. Perhaps the need is actually even greater. While we recognize, in other chapters, the attributes and value of other types of teaching, we would suggest that bedside teaching is a particularly critical type, in which residents should perhaps be most expert.

Residents may need to be particularly excellent bedside teachers because of the documented infrequency with which faculty approach the patient when teaching. (When we refer to bedside teaching, by the way, we include ambulatory patient-based experiences as well.) Anecdotal experience suggests that "modern" full-time faculty are rarely seen teaching with the patient. In one study, less than a quarter of attending round time was spent with the patient, and most of that was devoted to the demonstration of physical findings (Payson and Barchas, 1965). Collins *et al.* found that, in pediatric hospital teaching rounds, only 16 percent of the time was "actually spent at the bedside or with a patient present; and for at least half of that . . . the presence of the patient was not actually necessary to the discussion. In fact, most rounds tended to take place in the corridor, an area ill-suited to discussions of any type" (1978, p. 430). A study in 1964 noted in 25 percent of cases that the attending faculty member did not see the patient, either during or after ward rounds. (Reichsman *et al.*, 1964). Clearly, the supervising or chief resident has an important role to fill in taking the junior resident or medical student to the bedside or examination room, and junior residents fill a similar role specifically with medical students.

What are the advantages of teaching based upon the presence of the patient? Linfors and Neelon (1980, p. 1232-33) list three, to which we would add a fourth. They noted that 1) "the patient can be seen as an individual," *with* whom medical decisions are made, rather than *to* whom procedures and tests are applied, thus humanizing and personalizing medical care; 2) the presence of the patient helps the teaching process to be more participative, such that teachers and learners together have the collegial opportunity to understand the patient's problems and find ways to solve them; and 3) bedside teaching is the ultimate manifestation of the "physician" as "teacher," rather than as "lecturer," "discussant," or "consultant;" this role modeling behavior is critical to the student's professional development. The advantage we would add is that bedside teaching is essentially the only method in which the teacher has the opportunity to observe patient care skills directly and give immediate feedback. Thus, with reference to learning objectives, bedside teaching is the only way in which *evaluation* of *interviewing, physical examination,* and *psychomotor* skills can be done accurately and immediately.

Given these advantages, why does bedside teaching occur with such apparent infrequency? Linfors and Neelon note that a sort of "clinical entropy is dispersing learners from the bedside" (1980, p. 1231). They give five reasons for this. *First,* there is a false concern for the comfort and well-being of the patient. Several studies (Linfors and Neelon, 1980; Engel, 1971; Romano, 1941) actually show that the bedside teaching is not only *not* invasive or uncomfortable, but is usually a positive, reassuring, and comforting experience. We should note one study (we think poorly done) that purported to find an increased rate of death from myocardial infarction in patients recently visited on bedside rounds (Jarvinen, 1955). *Second,* some physicians feel that patients should not be involved at all in medical decision making, even through participation in bedside teaching. This "medical chauvinism" is clearly inappropriate in the current day. *Third,* some physicians (perhaps the same group as that described above) imagine that medical education should always consist of the direct transmission of knowledge from the active teacher to the passive learner. Clearly, bedside teaching can expand upon this limited view of learning to accomplish higher order learning objectives. *Fourth,* many teachers wish to limit their discussions to scientific data, particularly to the area in which they feel expert. Understanding and using the wealth of data generated for most patients can be overwhelming to both teacher and learner, and the presence of an additional complicating factor, a real live patient, can become the proverbial straw on the back of the educational camel. *Fifth,* many teachers fear they lack the necessary complex interactive skills to lead an elegant, erudite, and compassionate Oslerian-type discussion. In reality, as we shall show, this is not the case. The necessary skills are those which any experienced clinician should have: the ability to make the small, but critical, cognitive transitions from "knowing" to "doing" to "showing," and thereby follow the dictum of surgical education, "see one, do one, teach one." Residents can, and must, fill this role.

2. Active-passive Model

Bedside teaching is a form of preceptorship, in which the teacher is relatively more active and the student relatively more passive.

Figure Ie.
Active-passive Model for Bedside Teaching

	Active Teacher	Passive Teacher
ACTIVE LEARNER	Group Discussion	Tutorial
PASSIVE LEARNER	Lecture Preceptorship	

The teacher's active involvement in guiding the discussion, role-modeling attitudes, demonstrating psychomotor skills and procedures, and providing feedback are critical to the outcome.

3. Learning Objectives

As we have previously mentioned, while bedside teaching can *transmit knowledge* and stimulate *analysis* and *application,* its greatest use lies in accomplishing higher order objectives, such as *synthesis, evaluation,* modeling *affective* change, and teaching *psychomo-*

tor skills. Clinical problem solving can be taught in the patient's absence, such as in morning report, but a patient is required for the teacher to observe the learner collecting and synthesizing data, for the teacher to give direct feedback on the learner's performance, for the teacher to model and directly demonstrate patient care attitudes and professional behavior, and for the learner to see, and perform under supervision, certain examination or technical procedures. For example, previous studies have noted a remarkably high error rate by residents in the performance of routine physical examination (Weiner and Nathanson, 1976, Wray and Friedland 1983). No amount of lecturing or group discussion will correct these errors. Only bedside teaching, done with confidence and enthusiasm by an experienced clinician, has that potential.

4. Typical Activities

Bedside teaching can occur with equal success in both inpatient and outpatient settings. We think that the teaching techniques which follow could be applied in ward rounds supervised by either chief residents or faculty; in the teaching of bedside examination, diagnostic, or therapeutic procedures by senior or junior residents to other residents or medical students; in outpatient clinics, or other office settings, such as family practice centers, by residents of all levels; and in the teaching of procedures in the emergency room, operating room, and delivery room.

B. PRINCIPLES

Principle 1: ***Base all teaching on data generated by or about the patient.***

Bedside teaching has as its *only* purpose the teaching of knowledge, attitudes, and skills related directly to the patient who is present. This may seem obvious to, and therefore ignored by, some readers. The simplicity of this purpose may be missed by some bedside teachers, who then are unwittingly drawn into tangential discussions for which the patient's presence is only vaguely helpful. Also, some teachers may consider the patient to be someone whose purpose is to be impressed by the depth and breadth of the teacher's eloquent soliloquy on matters which may not always pertain to the patient's case. In both cases, the patient is confused, the learners embarrassed, and the value of the patient's presence is lost. We would suggest you keep in mind the advice of Sylvius, the 17th Century Chair of Medicine at Leiden, who wrote in 1664:

> "My method . . . (is to) lead my students by the hand to the practice of medicine, taking them every day to see patients in the public hospital, that they may hear the patient's symptoms and see their physical findings. Then I

> question the students as to what they have noted in the patients and about their thoughts and perceptions regarding the cause of the illnesses and the principles of treatment." (Linfors and Neelon, 1980, p. 1231).

In almost all cases, teaching should focus on history, examination, or laboratory data, or relate to a psychomotor skill being taught.

With regard to the conduct of bedside rounds, we recommend the problem-oriented approach initially described by Weed and modified by Hurst (1971). Hurst notes that the bulk of the patient presentation should *not* be made in the presence of the patient, but should adequately prepare the learners to benefit maximally from the time with the patient. "The time physicians and students spend with patients should be devoted entirely to the patient. Each patient is unique and what each says and reveals must be listened to and studied carefully" (Hurst, 1971, p. 464). This means that case presentations, either complete or partial, must be made succinctly, that all data bearing on a particular problem be presented together, that not all problems necessarily be discussed, that the presenter make clear an overview of the patient's situation, that the purpose of subsequently visiting the patient be made clear, and that time be allowed for questions between presentation and patient visit so that no confusion or ambiguity persists.

Remember always that "visits to the bedside can serve an important function, but they appear to do so only when they are conducted with a definite purpose in mind — e.g., to illustrate or confirm certain physical findings, to validate and expand on key points in the history, or to demonstrate appropriate methods of interacting with the patient" (Mattern *et al.,* 1983, p. 1131).

Principle 2: *Conduct bedside rounds with respect for the patient's comfort and dignity.*

We can make this point best by using Osler as an example. A description by one of his students indicated that Osler "would go to the patient's bed, stand (or sometimes sit in a chair) near the head of the bed at the patient's right side, give him a cheery greeting and, if he were a new patient, ask for his history. . . . After it had been commented on . . . and often added to and illuminated by Dr. Osler with accompanying pertinent remarks, the report of the physical examination was called for from the clinical clerk. . . . Usually Dr. Osler made some examination himself and demonstrated and discussed patient features, all the time mingling his discussion with remarks and explanations to the patient, so that he would not be mystified or frightened. . . . Often, patients whose cases had previously been discussed were passed over quickly, but Dr. Osler never failed to give some bright, cheering words to the patient" (Christian, 1949, pp. 81-82).

Several authors have noted the beneficial effect of bedside teaching to patients. Romano notes that "ward round teaching, when conducted tactfully and sympathetically . . . is not a traumatic emotional experience to patients, but educates and reassures them" (1941, p. 667). Linfors and Neelon found that 95 percent of patients saw bedside rounds as a positive experience, but that patients had several suggestions for improvement: "They wanted the attending physician to introduce himself, to state the purpose of bedside rounds, and to be sensitive to the need to translate technical terms. They also thought that the patient should receive advance notice of bedside rounds and that rounds should not be so long as to tire the patient" (1980, p. 1231). Hurst notes that the presenter, who should know the patient best, should visit the patient after rounds to clarify misunderstandings and relieve any anxieties created by rounds. Also, Hurst reinforces Osler's technique of leaving the bedside "with an optimistic statement of some sort even if it is no more than stating that the physicians caring for the patient are working diligently on the patient's problems" (1971, p. 1231). Showing due respect for the patient's comfort and dignity not only is necessary for good patient care, but also models excellent professional behavior by the teacher for the learners.

Principle 3: ***Always teach patient care skills at the level of the learner.***

Learners progress through four levels of sophistication as they learn new skills (*Personnel Journal,* 1974). Teachers must be aware of the level of sophistication at which a learner is currently functioning and match their teaching to that level. Teaching at a level of understanding greater or lesser than that of the learner is unproductive, frustrating, or both.

The four possible levels of understanding are:

1. unconsciously incompetent,
2. consciously incompetent,
3. consciously competent,
4. unconsciously competent.

Most learners are at level 1, where they do not even know what they do not know. Most teachers are at level 4, where they can "do it in their sleep." The teacher must join the learner, since the converse situation is impossible. For instance, in teaching a junior medical student how to draw an arterial blood specimen, the teacher would first make the learner aware of the technique's existence, the equipment required, the indications and contra-indications. The learner would then know what he/she does not know and be *consciously incompetent.* Proper demonstration and practice on models and patients would allow the learner to see and perform the procedure correctly, albeit with hesitation and anxiety, and thus become *consciously competent.* Hundreds of correct performances later, the learner would be *unconsciously competent.*

Many studies (Lamkin *et al.,* 1983; Stritter *et al.,* 1975) have been done of teacher behaviors that promote effective clinical learning, and all reach a similar conclusion with regard to teaching at the level of the learner. They show that teachers who, in addition to being competent and knowledgeable, are

- empathetic,
- compassionate,
- gentle,
- patient,
- interested in students and their needs,
- sensitive, and
- accessible to students

have the greatest success as clinical teachers. Being aware of the learner's past experiences, current needs, and current emotional state is critical to the success of teaching and role modeling patient care skills and behavior.

Principle 4: ***Use the methods of backward chaining or forward lengthening to teach sequential skills.***

Many medical or surgical procedures are actually a series of sequential steps, each of which must be performed correctly and in proper sequence. Examples include the physical assessment of the trauma patient, the mental status examination, and major surgical procedures. In order to teach these procedures effectively, it is important that they be broken into their discrete components rather than taught as an indigestible lump, and that one of two specific techniques be used to teach the sequence of steps.

In backward chaining, the *last* step is demonstrated and practiced *first,* so as to give learners a sense of the procedure's endpoint and outcome. Each preceding step is then demonstrated and practiced, followed in sequence by the latter steps already learned. By the time the first step in a 10-step sequence is learned, the last step has been performed 10 times. For example, in the repair of a midline perineal episiotomy, the attending could teach first the final stage of subcuticular skin closure, then add to that (on the next patient) the placement of deep interrupted sutures in the rectovaginal septum, and finally teach the first step of a running, locked suture in the vaginal mucosa.

Forward lengthening works just the opposite of backward chaining. The *first* step is demonstrated and practiced *first,* and subsequent steps are added until the final step is reached. Note that we emphasize demonstration *and* practice. The dictum "see one, do one, teach one" may be a bit light in the number of repetitions recommended, but the principle is correct.

Principle 5: ***Give feedback on current performance to improve future performance.***

One of the important learning objectives of bedside rounds, which cannot be as well achieved by some other teaching formats, is evaluation by the teacher of the learner, as well as by the learner of the material. The giving of feedback to the learner is a critical part of the teacher's job. Christian observed that Osler was particularly good at this. "His criticisms of students and their work were incisive and unforgettable, but never harsh or unkindly; they inspired respect and affection, never fear" (Christian, 1949, p. 82).

The characteristics of feedback that will contribute most to future improvement are that it be:

- as specifc as possible,
- positive when deserved,
- not demeaning when critical,
- understandable,
- about things that can be changed, and
- well timed.

Telling a surgical resident that he is not fit to be a butcher does little to improve future performance, nor does the common practice of evaluating students by writing comments on an evaluation form that will not be seen for months after a rotation ends. Our experience has shown that giving feedback that conforms to the above six characteristics can be remarkably easy for the teacher and remarkably valuable for the learner.

Chapter VII
THE CLINICIAN AS TEACHER

We began this book with the question, "Why should a resident be a good teacher?" We offered two answers. *First,* residents do a lot of teaching, and therefore ought to be good at it. *Second,* to teach is to learn twice. We now ask a related question, "Why should a practicing physician be a good teacher?" The second answer still applies. After a physician enters practice, continuing to teach actively is probably the surest stimulus to continuing to practice excellent medicine, whether one, ten, or twenty years after training. Also, as we have noted previously, as a resident you provide a great service to attending physicians by taking seriously your responsibility for teaching them. Interestingly, the first answer also applies to the practicing physician. As we all know, the origin of the word "doctor" is the word "docere," meaning "to teach." This function of the physician does not end with residency training. As a practicing physician, you will be called upon to teach other physicians in the clinical department of your private hospital, to teach ancillary hospital personnel and your office staff, to provide preceptorships to residents and medical students as a clinical faculty member of a nearby medical school, and even to speak on medical subjects to community and civic groups. Perhaps most importantly, you are a teacher in every patient encounter, since patient education is perhaps the physician's most important function. For these reasons, we offer this final principle to guide you in your future career as a teacher-clinician.

PRINCIPLE: ***The most important characteristic of a successful clinical teacher is creativity.***

Creativity is a notion whose clarity diminishes as its study intensifies. However, creativity in teaching can be described, to a large extent, by two characteristics: 1) the degree to which the teacher is novel, and 2) the degree to which the teacher is useful (Whitman, 1983). These two characteristics can be arranged in a 2 x 2 matrix, as shown in Figure II. As you can see, the teacher who is both novel and useful is *creative,* and therefore successful. The teacher who is novel, but not useful, is a *charlatan* who will entertain, but not edify. The teacher who is useful, but not novel, is a *pedantic bore* whose experience and intelligence will remain forever a secret. We welcome your suggestions for what to call a teacher who is *neither* useful nor novel. Unfortunately, we have all had experience with this unnamed creature.

Figure II.
A Model for Creativity in Teaching

	Novel	Not Novel
USEFUL	Creative Teacher	Pedantic Bore
NOT USEFUL	Charlatan	?

The key to being a successful teacher, then, is to learn behaviors that make you both novel and useful. Several studies have determined which teacher behaviors contribute most to successful learning. These can all be listed according to whether the teacher is novel or useful, and we have listed them in this way in Table I. It is unfortunate, but true, that the teacher who is *novel* is *enthusiastic, stimulating, compassionate,* and *accessible to students.* (We wish that *all* teachers were like this and these behaviors therefore not so novel). The teacher who is *useful* is *well organized, competent, practical, answers questions,* and *emphasizes comprehension over recall.* If we accomplish nothing else in this book, we urge that, before each teaching experience, you read and follow the lists of behaviors in Table I.

We will end with another story. A highly acclaimed artist was being awarded first prize at a prestigious art show for a large collection of excellent works. The judge asked the artist which of her several pieces she considered to be her very best. She replied that *none* of the pieces on display was her very best. The judge was surprised that the artist had not brought her best work to the show. She replied that it was because her best work had yet to be done.

Becoming an excellent teacher requires continual learning and improvement, and each of us has yet to do our best teaching. We hope this book has helped you improve your teaching skills so that *your* best teaching has yet to be done.

Table I
NOVEL AND USEFUL BEHAVIORS OF THE IDEAL CLINICAL TEACHER (3 Studies)

	Novel	Useful
(Irby, 1978)	1. enthusiastic 2. adept at interacting with learners	1. clear and well organized
(Lamkin *et al.*, 1983)	1. stimulating 2. empathetic 3. compassionate 4. gentle 5. feeling 6. patient	1. competent 2. organized 3. well read 4. practical
(Stritter *et al.*, 1975)	1. enthusiastic 2. provides constructive feedback 3. genuine interest in students 4. accessible to students 5. dynamic and energetic 6. explains lucidly	1. answers questions 2. explains actions and decisions 3. provides opportunities to practice technical and problem solving skills 4. summarizes major points 5. makes difficult concepts understandable 6. emphasizes comprehension over recall 7. competent 8. well prepared 9. emphasizes important points 10. discusses practical applications of subject

REFERENCES

1. Abrami, Phillip C., Leventhal, L. and Perry, Raymond P. "Educational Seduction." *Review of Educational Research* 1982; 52: 446-464.
2. Brown, Robert S. "Staff Attitudes toward Teachings." *Journal of Medical Education* 1970; 45: 156-158.
3. Bunnell, Kevin P., editor. 1980. *Continuing Medical Educators Handbook.* Colorado Medical Society.
4. Bogdonoff, Morton D. "A Brief Look at Medical Grand Rounds." *The Pharos* 1982; Winter: 16-18.
5. Change Magazine Press, 1978. *Guide to Effective Teaching.* New Rochelle, New York.
6. Collins, George F., Cassie, Josephine M., and Daggett, Christopher J. "The Role of the Attending Physician in Clinical Training." *Journal of Medical Education* 1978; 53: 429-431.
7. Christian, Henry A. "Osler: Recollections of an Undergraduate Medical Student at Johns Hopkins." *Archives of Internal Medicine* 1949; 84: 77-83.
8. Donald, Janet G., and Shore, Bruce M. 1977. "Student Learning and the Evaluation of Teaching." in *If Teaching Is Important . . .* edited by Christopher K. Knapper *et al.* Canadian Association of University Teachers.
9. Elstein, Arthur S., Shulman, Lee S., and Sprafka, Sarah A. 1978. *Medical Problem Solving.* Cambridge, Mass., Harvard University Press.
10. Engel, George L. "The Deficiencies of the Case Presentation as a Method of Clinical teaching." *New England Journal of Medicine* 1971; 284: 20-24.
11. Howe, Michael. 1977. *Adult Learning.* New York: Wiley Co.
12. Hurst, J. Willis "The Art and Science of Presenting a Patient's Problems." *Archives of Internal Medicine* 1971; 128: 463-465.
13. Ingelfinger, Franz J. "The Graying of Grand Rounds." *The New England Journal of Medicine* 1978; 299: 772.
14. Irby, David "Clinical Teacher Effectiveness in Medicine." *Journal of Medical Education* 1978; 53: 808-815.
15. Jarvinen, Klaus A. "Can Ward Rounds be a Danger to Patients with Myocardial Infarction?" *British Medical Journal* 1955; February 5: 318-320.

16. Lamkin B., Mygdal, W. K., and Hitchcock, M. "Perceptions of the Ideal Clinical Teacher: Views of Family Medicine Educators." Family Practice Faculty Development Center of Texas 1983; 4: 1-6.

17. Jewett, Leslie S., Greenberg, Larrie W., and Goldberg, Rhonda M. "Teaching Residents How to Teach." *Journal of Medical Education* 1982; 57: 361-366.

18. Knox, Alan B. "Helping Teachers Help Adults Learn." *Teaching Adults Effectively,* edited by Alan B. Knox. *New Directions for Continuing Education* 1980; 6: 73-100.

19. Lawson, Barbara K., and Harvill, Leo M. "The Evaluation of a Training Program for Improving Residents' Teaching Skills." *Journal of Medical Education* 1980; 55: 1000-1005.

20. Linfors, Eugene W., and Neelon, Francis A. "The Case for Bedside Rounds" *New England Journal of Medicine* 1980; 303: 1230-1233.

21. Machlup, Fritz. "Poor Learning from Good Teachers." *Academe* 1979; October: 376-380.

22. Mattern, William D., Weinholtz, D., and Friedman, Charles P. "The Attending Physician As Teacher." *New England Journal of Medicine* 1983; 308: 1129-1132.

23. McKusick, Victor A. "No Graying of Grand Rounds at Hopkins." *The New England Journal of Medicine* 1979; 300: 440.

24. Naftulin, Donald H., Ware, John E., Jr., and Donnelly, Frank A. "The Doctor Fox Lecture: A Paradigm of Educational Seduction." *Journal of Medical Education* 1978; 48: 630-635.

25. National Medical Audiovisual Center. 1976. *Storyboarding/Visualizing Virtues.* Atlanta: NMAC.

26. Osler, William "On the Need of a Radical Reform in our Methods of Teaching Senior Students." *The Medical News* 1903; 82: 49-53.

27. Payson, H. E., and Barchas, J. D. "A Time Study of Medical Teaching Rounds." *New England Journal of Medicine* 1965; 273: 1468-1471.

28. *Personnel Journal,* "Conscious Competency — The Mark of a Competent Instructor." July, 1974: 538-539.

29. Plaut, S. Michael. "Preparation of Abstracts, Slides, and Presentations." *Clinical Research* 1982; 30: 18-24.

30. Reichsman, Franz, Browning, Francis E., and Hinshaw, J. Raymond. "Observations of Undergraduate Clinical Teaching in Action." *Journal of Medical Education* 1964; 39: 147-163.

31. Romano, John. "Patients' Attitudes and Behavior in Ward Round Teaching." *Journal of American Medical Association* 1941; 117: 664-667.

32. Rubeck, Robert F., and Pratt, Daniel D. "Conducting Case-Based Discussions." *The Arizona Medical Educator* 1978; 8: November.

33. Russell, I. Jon. *et al., 1983.* "Effects of Three Types of Lecture Notes on Medical Student Achievement." *Journal of Medical Education* 1983; 58: 627-636.

34. Skinner, B. F., 1948. *Walden Two.* New York: The Macmillan Co.

35. Stritter, F. T., Hain, J. D., Grimes, D. A. "Clinical Teaching Reexamined." *Journal of Medical Education* 1975; 50: 876-882.

36. Weiner S., and Nathanson, M. "Physical Examination: Frequently Observed Errors." *Journal of American Medicine Association* 1976; 236: 852-855.

37. Whitman, Neal. "Teaching Problem-Solving and Creativity in College Courses." Research Currents, Eric Clearinghouse on Higher Education, National Institute of Education, Washington D.C., 1983.

38. Whitman, Neal. "Choosing and Using Methods of Teaching," *Performance and Instruction* 1981; 5: 16-19.

39. Whitman, Neal, and Schwenk, Thomas L. "A Handbook for Group Discussion Leaders: Alternatives to Lecturing Medical Students to Death." University of Utah School of Medicine, Salt Lake City, Utah 1983.

40. Wray, M. P., and Friedland, J. A. "Detection and Correction of House Staff Error in Physical Diagnosis." *Journal of American Medical Association* 1983; 249: 1035-1037.

University of Utah School of Medicine

Handbooks to Improve Medical Teaching

There is No Gene for Good Teaching: A Handbook on Lecturing for Medical Teachers

PREPAID	$6.00
POSTPAID	$7.00

A Handbook for Group Discussion Leaders: Alternatives to Lecturing Medical Students to Death

PREPAID	$6.00
POSTPAID	$7.00

Evaluating Medical School Courses: A User Centered Handbook

PREPAID	$10.00
POSTPAID	$12.00

Residents as Teachers: A Guide to Educational Practice

PREPAID	$6.00
POSTPAID	$7.00

Preceptors as Teachers: A Guide to Clinical Teaching

PREPAID	$6.00
POSTPAID	$7.00

Send orders or inquiries to . . .

Dr. Neal Whitman
Department of Family and Community Medicine
University of Utah School of Medicine
50 North Medical Drive
Salt Lake City, UT 84132
Telephone (801) 581-3614

PLEASE MAKE CHECKS TO UNIVERSITY OF UTAH.
POSTAGE AND HANDLING IS INCLUDED IN THE QUOTED PRICES.